It's All Relative

Praise for It's All Relative: One Family's Story of Kidney Disease

Thank you, Jennifer, for your wonderful book about how your family has dealt with PKD [polycystic kidney disease], through family and personal experience. There needs to be more books about PKD out there so people can understand this disease and how it touches everyone in the family both emotionally and physically. Thank you for sharing your story.
-- Patti M (Kidney Patient)

An intriguing glimpse into the challenges families face when dealing with life-altering health issues. Often these health issues are genetic with few alternatives or choices available. Jennifer Florax illustrates how her personal experiences can provide support, understanding and insight into persons experiencing a similar situation.

-- T. Cloake, P.Eng (Retired)

A good understanding of PKD and how it affects

the patient and their loved ones. This family journey should remind us how precious our health is!

-- Maria Spinelli-Tisi, Pharmacist

It's All Relative

ONE FAMILY'S STORY OF
KIDNEY DISEASE

Jennifer Florax

Disclaimer
The stories offered in this book are not a replacement for medical advice. This book is a simple sharing of stories, perspectives, challenges and homemade solutions, not based on medical evidence. Ensure you consult with your medical team for sound advice.

It's All Relative: One Family's Story of Kidney Disease
ISBN: 978-1-7383456-0-1
EISBN: 978-1--7383456-1-8

By Jennifer Florax

Copyright © 2024 by Jennifer Florax

All rights reserved. No part of this publication may be reproduced, distributed, or transmitted in any form or means, including photocopying, recording, or other electronic or mechanical methods, without the prior written permission of the author, except in the case of brief quotations embodied in critical articles and reviews and certain other non-commercial uses permitted by copyright law.

Cover Artwork provided by iStock https://www.istock-photo.com/

First Printing, 2024

To
Lily and Clarence
without them
there would be no
us

Contents

  2

Author's Note   3

Forward   5

Kidneys - the Organs   7

Symptoms of Kidney Disease   15

Welcome to our Family

Our Story   30

Donna   34

Roy   37

Jean   41

Heather   45

Jeffrey   53

Jennifer	66
Jeremy	74
Justin	88
End of the Story...sort of	91
Frequently Asked Questions	93
Acknowledgements	99
References	100
About The Author	103
Other books by Jennifer Florax	104

Through the vines

Through the vines, we are connected
Intertwining ever winding
Like the blood through our veins
Bestowing life through the vines

Starting as seed
New foliage, new beginnings
The vines grow
Finding their way

Support to the vines
Guiding toward the sun
Sometimes they trail, sometimes they burrow
Not perfect, but thriving in their way

Branching out, new vines grow
Spreading their leaves
New builds on old
Through the vines, still connected

Pulling away, coming together
Splitting off, yet still bound
Drifting away and starting anew
The pull of the roots brings us home

– by Jennifer Florax

Author's Note

I am not the author of every story in this narrative; I am merely a participant and conduit for the numerous voices and experiences. My family has generously provided their personal stories in this collaborative effort to provide some awareness and support for kidney disease. Kidney disease flies under the radar. It's not a "sexy" disease; it doesn't garner a lot of attention in the medical world, as far as I can tell. It's not visible to the naked eye. When you are sick, you may look somewhat tired, but there are no outward symptoms and nothing dramatic.

The point of this book is to offer a glimpse into kidney disease, specifically Autosomal Dominant Polycystic Kidney Disease (ADPKD). There are many different types of kidney disease, all with the same result: years of dialysis and then a transplant if you're lucky. My family and I have ADPKD galloping through our genes, and we thought to share our story and hopefully offer some comfort and support for anyone going through this disease. Each story shared is based on perspective. Some points and facts may be different, but that's okay. Our stories reflect us as individuals, which includes our emotions and viewpoints, making each tale valuable.

My family has a strong disposition for the disease, with many of us in varying stages of failure, with the lucky ones receiving a transplant. Many people with this disease suffer in silence. There are usually no outward, visible symptoms indicating that someone is sick. There also isn't a "normal" progression path for this disease. Every person has different symptoms and different combinations of symptoms. Though we are related, each family member has experienced different paths toward failure and differing emotions. I hope that by sharing our lived experiences and the similarities and differences of the illness, I can demonstrate how no two cases are alike. Throughout the collection, each person tells their story from their mindset. My family has mentioned how cathartic the process has been for them to share what they have been through and know that maybe their thoughts can help others.

There are more of us out there. Here is our story.

Forward

Kidney Disease. Renal Failure. More specifically, Polycystic Kidney Disease or PKD. You never know when it's going to strike. Or, in my family, you play the waiting game – not **if** it will strike, but **when**. The unfortunate reality with polycystic kidney disease is that there isn't anything you can do to prevent it. Once you start to fail, there is nothing you can do to stop it. You can watch your salt intake, manage your blood pressure and drink many gallons of water, but if the cysts decide to take over, control is taken out of your hands. Your kidneys can either slowly fail in a gradual decline or quickly tank in their function. You can also plateau and live a long time with a lower function. But sometimes, the disease will fluctuate the kidney's function measure to give a bit of false hope.

More debilitating than the actual failure is the waiting game. Waiting for your kidneys to fail, knowing that you are going to get sick, and then a lot sicker after that. Finally, you have the hope that dialysis will make you feel better to get back to a semblance of everyday life, but that brings on a whole new set of challenges.

Kidneys - the Organs

We all have two kidneys. Your kidneys are organs about the size of your fist, tucked just under your ribcage on either side of your body. Your body creates waste, and your kidneys filter out that waste and dispel it from your body in the form of urine. Each kidney has little tubes called ureters connecting the kidneys to the bladder (you only have one bladder). In filtering out waste products, the kidneys create balance within your body, balancing mineral content, regulating blood pressure, removing excess water, and stimulating red blood cell production. Your blood is filtered through your kidney several times daily, filtering about 200 quarts a day. We eliminate about two quarts daily, meaning we reabsorb around 198 quarts. Healthy kidneys are an essential part of overall health. When kidneys begin to fail, it impacts all aspects of your health.

Autosomal Dominant Polycystic Kidney Disease

In our family, we have what is called Autosomal Dominant Polycystic Kidney Disease. It's a lot of words and is hard to say. It also takes a lot of work to explain. Autosomal Dominant means inherited, meaning that at least one parent must have the abnormal gene to produce the polycystic kidney disease. The abnormal gene occurs even if the matching gene from the other parent is normal. The abnormal gene dominates. Because this is an inherited disease, there is a fifty percent chance of passing the disease on to your children, regardless of gender.

The PKD Foundation of Canada states that *Autosomal dominant polycystic kidney disease (ADPKD) is fluid-filled cysts that grow to enlarge in both kidneys, eventually leading to kidney failure. It is the fourth leading cause of kidney failure. More than fifty percent of people with ADPKD will develop kidney failure by age fifty.* The average size of a typical kidney is a human fist. Polycystic kidneys can get much larger, some growing as large as a football and weighing up to thirty pounds each. Imagine the space large kidney take up not to mention the extra weight the body takes on.

The PKD Foundation goes on to state: that unlike some genetic diseases, ADPKD does not skip a generation, approximately ten percent of the people diagnosed with ADPKD have no family history of the disease, with the disease developing as a spontaneous (new) mutation. Once a person has ADPKD, even through a spontaneous mutation, they have a fifty percent chance of passing it on to each of their children.

Interestingly, there are not any outward symptoms of being sick. It can even be pretty easy to ignore, particularly in the early stages of the disease. If you are one of the lucky ones who doesn't get stones, or ruptured cysts or your kidneys aren't overly large, then you will silently fail in function. However, if you have any of the above, your kidneys will frequently send messages to your body through pain and other symptoms that there is a problem. When there are no outward or visible signs of disease, others around you tend to forget or question why you are so tired or are sometimes skeptical in their belief that you are sick. An aunt once remarked that my eyes looked like *"two piss-holes in a snow bank."* Translation: I looked like shit from the fatigue!

There isn't any treatment, and there is no cure. You get sick, you wait to fail, you go on dialysis, then you wait for a transplant. There isn't much else you can do.

Treatments for Renal Failure

There are three types of dialysis: in-center hemodialysis, home hemodialysis, and peritoneal dialysis.

A hospital or health care center nurse administers the in-center hemodialysis. Before you reach this stage, you must have a fistula created in a major vein. This fistula is basically the 'plug-in' for the tubes to clean your blood. The simplest explanation is your blood is pulled through a tube into a machine that scrubs all the waste out of your blood, and the cleaned blood is put back in your body with another tube.

Home hemodialysis is the same, but you do it in the comfort of your home. A healthcare team will help set you up, and there is always support a phone call away. You will need a connection to distilled water; regular old tap water won't work. This method means you don't have to travel to a hospital a few times a week, but you have to be able to hook yourself up to the machine.

Peritoneal dialysis makes use of the existing membranes within your body. All humans have a peritoneal cavity, a space within the abdominal wall, the pelvic cavity and the diaphragm. The membrane layer acts as a filter to screen out the body's waste. Before peritoneal dialysis is started, a tube is inserted into the mid to lower abdomen, feeding into this cavity and tucked just under the skin until needed. This surgery needs to heal before you can use the tube. Once you start dialysis, a special fluid is gravity-fed into the cavity. You carry this fluid around until your scheduled drain. While the fluid is in there, it cleans your blood. You empty the cavity and 'dirty' fluid through the same tube and gravity drain, then fill it with clean fluid. This process can be done manually four to five times per day. Or a machine will cycle this through you during the night.

Kidney patients usually have a choice of treatment, however, sometimes they do not. It all depends on the current state of your health. Unfortunately, there are times when one method will work and others won't, meaning you may have to switch dialysis methods. The hemodialysis generally does a better job of giving you a good clean but is physically hard on a person and may require some recovery time between treatments. The peritoneal may be easier on the body and allow some flexibility with life, but it may not clean your blood as efficiently as hemodialysis does.

Once you are on dialysis, you are then placed on the transplant list. The all-important "LIST." Theoretically, you move up the list in priority order or first come, first served. But it doesn't always work like that. Matches must be found; just because one is at the top of the list doesn't mean you are next up. The transplant team looks for the best fit for the available kidney. Best fit means that the transplant team will call in three or four people who fit on paper and retest them to check if they could be the best match. Then it's the waiting game. If you get the call that you are the match, it's like winning the lottery–you could be the winner or have to wait some more.

One can receive a transplant in one of two ways. A deceased donor has donated their organs or a live donor, meaning a family member or friend who matches you, will donate their kidney to you. A live donor means the donor and recipient undergo surgery simultaneously. One is having a kidney removed, and the other is getting a new kidney. The new kidney in either method is usually placed on your right side, tucked under your intestines. The non-working kidneys are not removed as that is considered unnecessary surgery.

Sometimes patients go public with their need for a kidney. But unfortunately, their need only raises the profile for that one person and then the desire to help disappears. There are so many others out there. A living donor is a very selfless thing to do but it could be putting the person who donates at risk as it's not an easy surgery to recover from. A live donor has about a six to eight-week recovery time. While it is terrific that someone was helped by going public, there isn't any sustained awareness of the need for kidneys.

Symptoms of Kidney Disease

The interesting thing about polycystic kidneys is that no one has all the same symptoms. Some have very few symptoms, and others have many signs something is wrong. The symptoms can be managed if you care for yourself and pay attention to what your body tells you. But the knowledge that you are going to continue to get sicker is not something that can be treated. It's like a great weight sitting on you, that no matter what you do, you are going to be sicker than you are right now.

Some of the symptoms or side effects of polycystic kidneys are kidney stones, fatigue, nausea, restless legs, ruptured cysts, infections, headaches and possibly others.

Pain

Any pain that you have is real. Doctors tend to tell you that you shouldn't have any pain and that there is no pain with kidney disease. However, trust in yourself. The way you feel is valid. The kidney sometimes feels swollen; picture a writhing, pulsating, contorted mass (kind of like The Blob) trying to push its way out of your body between your ribs. If you're a woman, wearing a bra can be painful. It sometimes feels like your bra is a boa constrictor, tightening around you, cutting off circulation and generally adding to the discomfort.

With the growth of your kidneys, logic dictates that there is only so much room in your torso. People are not built to contain kidneys three or four times bigger than they should be. It can feel like your kidneys are absorbing all the extra room, pushing on your other organs. Your stomach is compressed by the bigger kidneys taking up the available space making you feel full faster than normal contributing to nausea.

I've spent a fair bit of time trying to think of how to describe what this feels like. I encourage anyone without the disease to try the following scenario; it will help with some understanding of what a polycystic kidney disease (PKD) patient goes through.

Get up at about 3:30 am., but don't drink coffee (sorry for the extra punishment). A few hours later, when you are good and tired, tie a ball of yarn about the size of a baseball to your sternum–right at the mid-section of your ribs. But not a nice soft ball of yarn, but reroll it so it's nice and hard. Then, take some more rerolled yarn of varying sizes, some big and small put them in a plastic bag, and tie them to your stomach. I suggest a good ten or twelve balls of yarn. Ensure all your yarn is good and tight against your full abdomen. Then, find a small bag and fill it with rocks. Don't pick nice, smooth ones; make sure they are jagged and pointy. Place it under your shirt against where one of your kidneys is located. Secure it in place as best you can. Now get comfortable! While you are trying to get comfortable, imagine a knife sticking you in between the ribs every once in a while. You probably can't go to work or do anything during this get-up, but imagine you have to. Imagine that you have to function every day with all of these sensations. This is a day in the life of what a PKD patient feels.

Nausea

Nausea seems to come from the pressure of your kidneys pushing on the other organs. Or it could simply be a side effect of the buildup of toxins. Sometimes, certain foods don't sit right. In my case, the nausea comes and goes if I eat sugar. Each person will need to experiment with their nausea to eliminate the foods that may trigger it. But it changes; what sat well before may change the next day. There doesn't appear to be a medical reason for this symptom. One day, the food items are just fine and the next, you're heaving over the toilet. And sometimes, it's just random or can accompany other things like kidney stones. In my experience, kidney stones do seem to trigger nausea.

I've noticed that overeating seems to bring on a good round of nausea as well. For example, you're at a big family holiday dinner with so many choices, and your eyes are bigger than your stomach, and you try a bit of everything. It could be the combination, but most likely, it is the volume. There isn't enough room for food, particularly if your kidneys are big.

Kidney Stones

Kidney stones are just that: stones. A stone can form from salt or protein and potassium waste products. The most common type of kidney stone is a calcium oxalate stone. Most kidney stones are formed when oxalate, a byproduct of certain foods, binds to calcium as urine is being made by the kidneys. Having kidney stones feels like someone is shoving a serrated knife in your back and twisting it. Accompanying this pain are nausea and an urgent need to pee. The pain can take the breath out of you. Sometimes, blood can also be found in your urine because the stones have little jagged edges that slice into the urinary tract as they pass through. When the stones finally pass, it is such a relief, almost instant. Unfortunately, you can get used to the pain and don't even realize when some of them pass.

Fatigue

There's not much to do about the fatigue, it is unavoidable. Although difficult, make yourself do something: go for a walk, do your hobby, or do anything physical. You will feel like shit at the time, but it does help. A good nap also does wonders. The fatigue can suddenly hit, you may feel fine for one minute, and then you are so tired it's a wonder you don't fall over. Take the time to nap. Though it feels like you are sleeping your life away, at least you can function for another few hours. The draggy feeling also impacts the brain fog, which I will discuss shortly. It's a vicious cycle of trying to get enough sleep to function but being unable to sleep because of restless legs (a strong, uncontrollable urge to move the legs). Then, the brain fog gets worse. Any pain you have also contributes to your fatigue, it's like your body uses fatigue to protect you from some of the pain. With your body constantly trying to protect you from the pain, muscles tense up and become a cycle of more pain. Sometimes, you can almost feel impaired because you are so tired. I had never felt fatigue like this, even worse than the sleepless nights of early parenthood.

Restless Legs

Restless legs only seem to happen when you try to sleep. It generally starts in the evening as you are trying to relax. It's not pain but more of an odd sensation. Your legs move of their own accord. The sensation is similar to cold water running through the veins in your legs with an involuntary desire to move them accordingly. If you try to make it stop, it feels even worse or you simply can't. Sometimes, you spend the night wandering the house, then you are so tired that functioning becomes a problem, and then you do it all again the next night.

Some preventative tips that I've learned through experimentation, but they don't always work:

- Going for a walk seems to help stimulate the muscles ahead of time
- Stretching: same as going for a walk
- Massage: seems to get the muscles to calm down, at least for a short time

- Creams: some magnesium creams help a bit, and they are topical, so they don't interfere with other medication
- Ice cubes on your legs: It appears to calm the muscles down
- Limiting caffeine in the afternoon helps reduce the potential for restless legs
- Discuss with a doctor about medication that helps to limit the movement.

Brain Fog

Losing words, not processing information, staring blankly at someone and wondering what the hell they are saying to you—all part of brain fog. If you're a woman and hitting a particular stage of life, you are in for a double whammy of brain fog. Brain fog isn't your imagination; it is happening. It is frustrating and quite scary. Your brain is kind of a vital organ that you need for everyday life. What I call *'losing your brain'* can be more terrifying than kidney disease. You need your brain for function, and if you're losing it, then what happens?

I don't know the entire cause, but I assume

that fatigue plays a role in some brain fog. Or the simple fact that you don't have working kidneys to flush the toxins out of your body. For the brain fog, you need to find some strategies to help you with your memory. For me, I moved off of the electronic note-taking and went back to pen and paper. Physically writing things down, or developing shorthand notes helps jog the memory, particularly in the workplace.

Itchy skin

With PKD, sometimes, your skin is a little on the dryer side and can be flaky and scratchy. Itching can be localized to a small area of the body or it could be an all-encompassing itch over the entire body. I am assuming that some of this is due to some dehydration issues. But it could also be the toxin build-up from your kidneys not doing their job. Drinking more water and using a scentless lotion with aloe can help. Scent generally has other agents in it that will dry your skin more.

Infections

Infections within the urinary tract and bladder are more common in women than in men. Kidney infections are not overly common, but they do happen. The challenge begins when your body tells you there is an infection but doesn't show up on any standard test. In my experience, every infection shows up a little differently than the previous one, presenting with different symptoms or very few symptoms. In general symptoms of infection are as follows: increased urination, the urge to pee, burning pee, nausea, cramps, pain in the flank and sometimes headaches. A good doctor who believes in you, even without a positive test, is your saving grace.

Home remedies

Through my experimentation and experiences, here are a few tips you can try at home to relieve symptoms:

- Heating pad: helps to ease some of the pain in your back; the hotter, the better. It relaxes the tense muscles surrounding the kidney area.
- Ice Water: Lots of ice and cold water help with nausea. Using a straw also seems to help regulate water intake, so you don't make the nausea worse by drinking too fast.
- Ginger Gravol: It doesn't make you sleepy, helps with nausea, and doesn't interfere with other medications that you might be on.
- Ginger Ale: Flat, plain ginger ale. Pour a glass of ginger ale and stir with a spoon until it is almost flat can help with nausea.
- Curl on your side in the fetal position

and don't be afraid to cry: the position eases the pain, and crying relieves the stress from the pain.
- Place pressure on your back: Some pressure feels good. Ball up a sweater, position it where the pain is and ease into it, a pillow works or anything pliable enough to form as needed.
- Tea: Mint, peppermint or green tea helps with nausea and chamomile or sleepy time tea helps at night. Try to drink it without any sugar or milk, just plain.

These home remedies worked for me but they may not work for others. Experiment with your limitations, but make sure you don't overdo it. Don't do anything outside of your regular healthcare treatments and always consult with your healthcare team.

Welcome to our Family

Over the last few decades, medical research has learned new things about this disease. Not just the medical research, improvements in technologies and transplant success rates. What we knew forty years ago is different than what we know today. In the past, people didn't have the same access to information that they do today, nor did they think to question the doctors as we do now.

Today, we have different information that supports our healthcare decisions. Patients have access to research and other opinions that are continually evolving. We are encouraged to learn and partner with our doctors for our healthcare needs.

Now that the technical aspects of polycystic kidney disease are out of the way, we can get to the real story–the people story. Many in my family have been impacted by polycystic kidney disease. Every one of us has a slightly different experience, slightly different memories and perspectives and varying reactions to the influence polycystic kidney disease has had on our lives. As you read through our stories you'll see that age, time, and experience play a factor in how we have perceived the diagnosis and our interactions with other family members through this wild ride.

Each person who has shared their story has different ways of coping with the diagnosis of polycystic kidney disease. Physical symptoms vary widely between patients and so too do the emotional impacts. The riotous swings in emotions illustrate how this disease impacts everyone differently. As you continue this journey with us, keep in mind that you are reading about real people with real-world experiences. Each person has chosen to share their path or portions of their path, detailing their memories, emotions and personal thoughts. As you read these stories, note that each is written in the first person. An organizational chart is provided to help guide the reader.

Our Family Connections

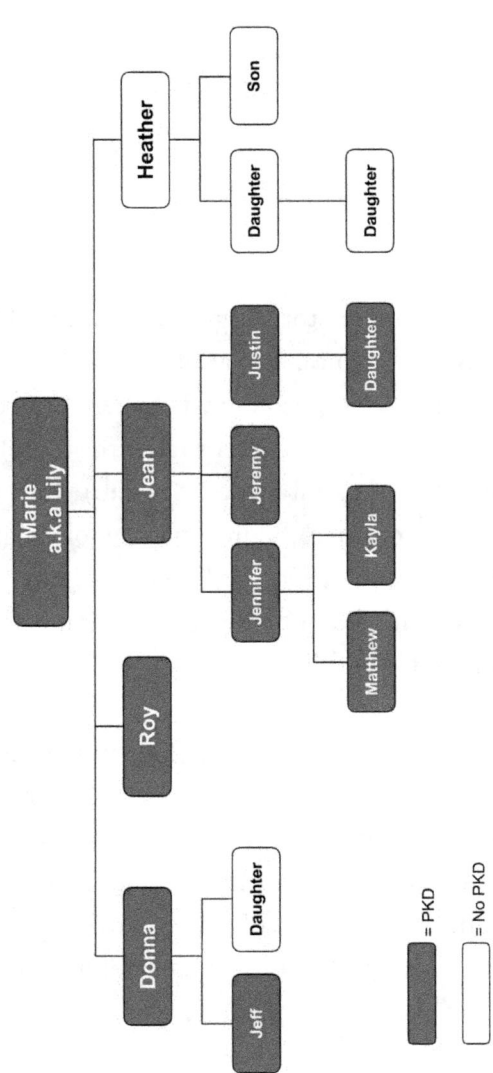

Our Story

Our family story begins with Marie Elizabeth Ransbottom (nee. Lacombe), a.k.a. Lily. She was born on May 9, 1926, in Kerobert or Scott, Saskatchewan (she was never sure of the town) to Fred and Mary Lacombe (nee. Schwab). Lily was the youngest of three children, with an older sister and an older brother. To our knowledge, Lily's parents and siblings did not have any serious medical issues and lived long full lives.

Lily was born with one kidney that happened to be polycystic. As per the research, Lily appears to have spontaneously developed the mutated gene to end up with Autosomal Dominant Polycystic Kidney Disease (ADPKD), eventually passing this gene on to her children, grandchildren, and great-grandchildren. Interestingly, the gene did not pass on to all of her children. Three of the four have the disease and have passed it on. The fourth does not appear to have the disease, nor have passed the disease to the children.

Unfortunately for Lily, her diagnosis was well beyond the progression of the disease. She was sick most of her life with a variety of ailments, including fatigue, mental health issues, headaches, vomiting for no apparent reason and bowel challenges. Lily also always had a distended belly, giving the appearance of pregnancy. The assumption is that the growth and large kidney pushed her belly outwards. She spent a lot of her adult life being exhausted and sick without knowing why. She was treated for many different potential issues through the process of elimination, including gallstones. As if being ill was not enough, life threw her another curve ball in the form of a lump in her breast. In those days, they didn't do much investigation or treatment; they simply did a mastectomy. Unfortunately, all the symptom treatments provided to Lily were hard on the kidneys, which we imagine made things worse for her.

Lily's diagnosis of Polycystic Kidney Disease was finally received in 1976; knowledge and testing were not as accurate as it is now. By the time her kidney disease was discovered at age 49, Lily had five percent of her kidney function. Due to her place of residence and available medical knowledge at the time, there weren't always doctors available to support or help manage her symptoms. Once Lily reached the point of failure and needed dialysis, the family had some decisions to make.

Living in a small town made access to doctors and dialysis extremely difficult. Lack of access to treatment meant that Lily, her husband, Clarence (born April 26, 1908, died April 8, 1994), and her youngest daughter had to move to Edmonton, Alberta, to access dialysis, kidney specialists and more accessibility to the hope of a kidney transplant. The entire family had to be uprooted and adjusted to access treatment. In the 1970s, there was only hemodialysis and only in larger cities. Peritoneal treatment was not available until much later and was not an option for Lily. Their only choice was to move close to a major hospital to be able to receive hemodialysis three times per week.

Interestingly, Lily's three oldest children were tested to see if they were a match to become a living donor. Doctors were surprised to learn that the three they tested also had the same kidney disease, but not as progressed. We assume that research had not made the genetic connection at the time.

Lily passed away on January 27, 1981, in Valleyview, Alberta. She was 54.

Donna

> *Donna is the oldest child of Lily and Clarence, her son is Jeffrey and she has a daughter. Her sisters are Jean and Heather and her brother Roy. As Donna has passed, the author has written this story.*

Donna, the oldest child of Lily and Clarence, was born March 1, 1951. She married Richard and had a son and a daughter. We lost Donna in a car accident in July 1992. We don't know how she was feeling and we have no insight into her specific health as she didn't appear to share those details with anyone. However, she did have some kidney stones that we were aware of. Donna had been having some heart troubles before the accident, and it is unclear if that was related to kidney disease. We do know that she passed polycystic kidney disease on to one of her two children. We found out after she had passed that she wasn't far away from needing dialysis.

I remember my Aunt Donna's hugs; they were all-encompassing. She hugged with her whole being. She also needed everything around her clean. I remember her always having a damp wash cloth in a plastic bag in case of a dirt emergency, I guess. One memory I'll share is of my cousin, brother and I were playing outside. I think it had rained a few days earlier, and there were large puddles of water all over the yard. Imagine dirt potholes filled with water. The three of us decided kicking all the water and mud out of the puddle would be pretty fun. It was the only time I saw Aunt Donna completely lose her temper with us. The three of us had mud from head to toe. Aunt Donna chucked us all in the bathtub and had to wash all our clothes. I remember sitting quietly, wrapped in a towel until our clothes were clean; unfortunately for my brother and me, that was the moment when our parents came to pick us up. We were all quite young, and I don't remember what happened after that, but I can imagine the conversation they would have had!

Roy

> Roy is the second-born and only boy of Lily and Clarence. Donna, Jean and Heather are his sisters.

When I think back, my mom was first diagnosed with polycystic kidney disease sometime between 1973 and 1975. She had been sick for a while without knowing the real cause. Mom's primary diagnosis of acute renal failure was finally received in December 1975. All of her older children were tested as possible kidney donors for Mom, except for Heather, who was too young to be considered a possible donor. When we were tested as potential donors, all three of us older children were found to have polycystic kidney disease as well. There was mention that there may or may not be further problems for us down the road. Not much more information than that was provided.

After Mom passed, there wasn't much conversation among the family regarding our potential to be diagnosed with the same disease. When I was first diagnosed, I was dismayed, but I thought of other families that had to deal with something like any hereditary issue and figured if they could, we could too. I already had heart issues that I was dealing with, so the thought of another disease was put out of my mind. In 1989, I started developing kidney stones, then more stones a few years later. By 1996, my kidney function was beginning to be monitored until around 2003, when I had my third aortic valve replacement.

Around 2004, I was told I needed to consider my dialysis options as I may need to start down that road. Still, that decision was then postponed to September 2005, when I started peritoneal dialysis. I chose peritoneal dialysis as opposed to hemodialysis as it offered more freedom. I was cattle farming at the time and did fluid transfers wherever I was to keep to the schedule. Sometimes this meant doing the transfers in the cab of my truck, or even in the furnace room at the cattle auction market. I did my dialysis four times per day.

I was not doing well with the dialysis, and my healthcare team wanted to adjust my treatment to a different method. With my current peritoneal method, I was putting in four litres of fluid with only three litres coming out, leaving me with a condition similar to that of a steer with a water belly (accumulation of urine under the belly skin in the abdominal cavity).

I was shocked to receive a call just after midnight on January 2, 2007, as I completed my night transfer using the peritoneal system. At first, I thought it was a scam or some kind of joke. I didn't recognize the caller's voice, but the person identified themselves as a doctor with more details than a scammer would have. Then I thought I might be dreaming, but I was wide awake. I was told to be at the University of Alberta Hospital in Edmonton by 6:00 a.m. for a potential transplant. By 5:00 p.m. that night, I was told to have a shower as I was getting the new kidney.

My advice to others with the same disease is to stick to the plan, listen to your nephrologist and hope for a transplant.

Jean

> *Jean is the third child of Lily and Clarence. Her sisters are Donna and Heather and her brother, Roy. Her children are Jennifer, Jeremy and Justin.*

My memories from the time I was nine years old were of my mom always being sick and often having headaches and going to the doctor without any results or reasons for why she was ill. We didn't find out what was wrong until her kidney function was working at five percent—the toxin build-up and being sick for so long affected her mental health as well.

Cysts were discovered on my kidneys at age twenty-three. I honestly never thought about the cysts or my kidneys at the time. I had small children to care for and simply accepted the cysts for what they were. When my kidneys started to fail, I never really had any symptoms. I was tired leading up to the diagnosis but didn't know the reason. Finding out that this disease was genetic, I felt guilty and a little bitter for passing it on to my kids.

Just like my mom, I'm from a small town with minimal access to treatment. I had to move to Edmonton, Alberta, a bigger city, to increase my chances of receiving a transplant. Another life had to be uprooted because of this disease.

I elected to do peritoneal dialysis, and it went much better than expected. This method of treatment allowed me to continue working and going places because I could take it with me. Due to infections related to the peritoneal dialysis I was on hemodialysis for a short time, and it was hell. My body had trouble adjusting to this form of dialysis. I felt swollen in between treatments so the team would increase the concentration of solution, then too much was taken off and I would pass out. I swore if I had to do it again, I wouldn't; I would let nature take its course.

After having hemodialysis for only six weeks, I gained so much respect for others in my family who had to be on this treatment method for three or four years-especially my mom. She did it in the mid to late 1970s. The dialysis machines then looked much cruder than today, and she only had a folding chair to sit on. Plus, she had to ride the bus to and from the hospital by herself when Dad couldn't take her, sitting, connected to the dialysis machine for five hours. Yet she never complained about it; she took it in stride. She passed away from a brain aneurysm caused by kidney failure. At the time, no one knew that the two issues were connected.

When I received the call that I had a match for a transplant, I was shocked; not believing it was true. My daughter drove me to the hospital late at night for the blood work. That was when I learned that I was one of three people that may be a match for this kidney. The nurses took sixteen tubes of blood out of me–then sent us home. I waited at home, too keyed up to sleep. The hospital called around 2:00 a.m. to tell me the kidney was mine and to get to the hospital. At this point, I was scared, of what I didn't know. But I arrived at the hospital at 3:30 a.m. and received the transplant around 8:00 p.m. that night. It was a long time waiting, worrying, and wondering what would happen during the surgery.

My advice to others is not to dwell on the disease. Don't worry or stress about it; stress can and will affect kidney function. Take everything day by day, and you will get through it.

Heather

> *Heather is the youngest child of Lily and Clarence, she has a daughter and a son. Her sisters are Donna and Jean, and her brother Roy.*

My mom was sick as far back as I can remember. It was always something different, but, as we later learned, all her health issues could be attributed back to her kidney disease. She was born with only one functioning kidney, and it was polycystic. The other just never developed.

She was treated for many things, such as gallstones (which I don't believe she had) and depression, among other things. She had a complete hysterectomy in 1969, which wreaked havoc on her hormones, so she was given medication (not sure what; she just called them her "nerve pills"). She was advised by one physician, to start smoking cigarettes (menthol, mind you, let's not go crazy here) to "calm her nerves." It is clear how far medicine has evolved since then.

The summer of '69 stands out because she slept a lot, and my older sisters cared for me. I remember my sister, Donna, being around the most as she was eighteen that year and had just graduated high school. I'm pretty sure being stuck with a three-year-old was not how she saw her first summer of freedom going.

Mom was diagnosed with kidney disease in 1976 when her kidney function had dropped to less than five percent. However, her health had been rapidly deteriorating since approximately 1973, when a new family doctor began treating her for the aforementioned gallstones but did not run any other tests that I know of. She finally became so ill that they had to send her to Edmonton by ambulance, and she just never came home. My Dad did, and he told me they were moving to the city so Mom could get the treatment she needed. I was to go and live with my sister, Jean and her husband and a new baby who was not even a year old yet. He told me it was because they didn't want to pull me out of school. It must have been early in the fall, and school had just started because I'm pretty sure I stayed with Jean and John for about nine or ten months. I knew my parents thought they were doing what was best for me, but I remember feeling somewhat abandoned and then guilty for feeling that way. After raising two kids of my own and on my own, I do realize Dad had a lot on his plate with a sick wife, having to pack up and move in a hurry. He had just bought a house that we hadn't even taken possession of yet and had to ensure it had good tenants since we wouldn't be moving in for an undetermined amount of time. On top of everything going on, he was nearly 70 years old when all this happened.

Since her kidney could no longer do its job, she had very high levels of toxins in her system, which can harm one's mental health. What that meant for her was a stint in the psychiatric ward. I'll never forget that she was in hospital around Christmas. I'm not sure what year, but it must have been 1976 when she was first diagnosed. I remember visiting and being afraid of her, thinking, *"Why was my mom behaving so strangely? Why were all the other patients acting weird? Why did the nurses on this ward wear street clothes rather than nurses' uniforms?"* I had so many questions. My Dad and siblings tried their best to answer them. I think it was my brother Roy who told me that the sight of nurses' uniforms could upset some of the patients. I didn't get it. Mom had seemed to regress into the past, thinking my sisters were her sister, she had only one, so I can only assume she saw Donna and Jean separately. Anything else may have been more than she could take. She thought that my brother Roy was her brother, and my Dad was her Dad. I don't think she noticed me at all.

In this hospital, everyone got lumped together regardless of their diagnosis. There was another young patient who could play the piano beautifully, which calmed Mom so much when he played Wooden Heart. That is one pleasant memory of that time that I guess I clung to, and the nurses let me zoom up and down the hallway in the wheelchairs, they knew I was bored and felt bad for me, I suppose.

During all of this, they found a lump in one of Mom's breasts. They [the doctors] said they were going to do a biopsy, and while she was under the anesthetic, they decided to just skip ahead to the mastectomy as a "precaution." I don't think it was ever determined if she had breast cancer for sure. She was just fifty years old and would only live another four years. I have been getting annual mammograms since long before I would have been a candidate had I not had a family history of breast cancer. Since I'm not sure it is actually in our family history, it has never sat well with me that I've been exposed to so much radiation-not to mention the inconvenience and discomfort of the appointments themselves.

All in all, the medical community failed my mother. My parents, especially my mom, put all their faith in the doctors and other medical professionals because that was what their generation did. You trusted the people with degrees.

I don't have polycystic kidney disease like the rest of my family. I don't remember my siblings being diagnosed, as I was only nine or ten. I just always knew they had the genetic potential for kidney failure. So, I don't remember thinking anything of it as a child. I just grew up with the knowledge that they all had polycystic kidneys. What that meant, however, was not a formed thought. It was always something I knew about them like they had brown eyes or curly hair. It didn't hit me until I was an adult.

I did not have my kidneys checked until I was in my early thirties when my family doctor learned of our history. He told me I did not have the disease and, more importantly, that I would NEVER have it (he could safely say this due to my age at the time I was checked). My siblings had already been tested in case one was a potential match to donate a kidney to Mom. I wasn't tested at the time because I was too young to be a donor, and then I guess it just wasn't crucial with everything else going on.

Knowing I didn't have polycystic kidney disease was a relief at first. Then, my focus was on my kids and getting them checked, and they were both fine, thankfully. Then I remember wondering why it skipped me. Was I adopted or switched at birth? Then there was so much guilt that I was okay, guilt in my relief that my kids were okay, but the other grandchildren and possibly great-grandchildren were not. I felt guilty about having only one kidney to offer, and so many loved ones who would eventually need a transplant, and guilt because I was too scared to be a donor. I also had to consider that with so many family members in need, I could be a match for more than one of them. My kidney would go to the first one who needed it the most. What if that family member didn't care for themselves and the kidney got rejected? What a waste that would be. I did not want to go down that road.

My advice to others is not to beat yourself up because you were spared, and don't feel pressured to donate an organ. All surgical procedures, even the most routine ones, have the potential to be dangerous, and a living donor procedure is not routine. I don't think anyone should feel pressured to donate or feel bad if they are afraid to or don't want to.

There appears to be a rising need for organ donation. It feels like for the organs that living donors can donate, it is a societal assumption that if we "can" donate, we "should." I've read stories where strangers donated a kidney or part of their liver to someone in need. Then I feel guilty again. I wonder if they thoroughly understand what they are signing up for. I would hope they do, but it's not as simple as donating a pint of blood or some bone marrow.

My uncle had six children, five of whom are diabetic. I am pretty close with one of my cousins, and I once asked her if she thought her sister, who does not have diabetes, ever felt guilty. She said, *"I certainly hope not. I hope she feels grateful"*. Though not entirely the same because she can't do anything to cure or help her siblings who live with the disease. However, hearing this did help me to gain some perspective on my situation.

Once I am gone, all my organs can be harvested, should they be viable. But for now, I have decided to keep the ones I have.

Jeffrey

> *Jeffrey is the oldest grandchild of Lily and Clarence. His mother is Donna. He has one sibling.*

My memories of Grandma's dialysis experience are vague and supplemented with second-hand, after-the-fact information. I was still very young, so all I had at the time was a vague idea that something was wrong with Grandma and that she had to spend a lot of time in the hospital. I've learned since then that Grandpa, Grandma, and their young daughter moved to Edmonton from Valleyview in 1976 because there were no dialysis facilities nearby. That's understandable because dialysis was still in its formative era; the family must have considered themselves fortunate that the University of Alberta Hospital [Edmonton, Alberta] had the necessary facilities. A quick Google search informed me that home-based hemodialysis and peritoneal dialysis existed in the mid-1970s. However, I don't know if Grandma considered either of those options or if those programs were available in northern Alberta then.

I do remember that I loved the trips to Edmonton to see my Grandpa, Grandma, and Aunt, who was only seven years older than me and still a child herself. For some reason, my young mind considered their home some kind of suburban paradise.

This may have been because the family had access to cable TV with American programming we couldn't get on our two channels in Sunset House, Alberta (the farm community where we lived). That meant Saturday morning cartoons, which excited me to no end. What can I say? I was only a child.

Grandma received a kidney transplant in 1979, and shortly after that, the family moved back to

Valleyview, Alberta. I still had little idea of the exact nature of her illness, but I gathered that something good had happened to make Grandma better. Of all the things that stood out to me, though, was a kidney-shaped sticker on the refrigerator door that had something to do with the Kidney Foundation. That remained my mental image of a kidney for a very long time.

My final memories of Grandma revolved around her staying at our place for about a week in January 1981, shortly before her death. Grandma was always friendly but seemed particularly friendly and attentive towards me during this time. There's a snapshot in my mind in which I'm sitting on the living room couch. Grandma is at the kitchen table, looking at me directly and smiling. There are no words- just a smile. It remains to this day my most treasured memory of my grandmother.

Although I heard the words "kidney" and "disease" mentioned a lot within the family, they never really registered with me until Mom and Dad decided to proactively screen me for polycystic kidney disease at the age of nine. I remember at least two instances of having to fast for two days with nothing but Jell-O and ice cream to eat. It may sound like a kid's dream, but I quickly found neither quelled my hunger. Both times, I was rewarded for my sacrifice with a post-doctor appointment breakfast at Uncle Nicky's -- a favourite diner in High Prairie, Alberta.

The process concluded with a week-long stay at the University Hospital in Edmonton in December 1982. I have fond memories of that stay: the nurses were very friendly, and I became friends with my roommate because of our love of comic books, movies, and video games.

I think I was so busy having fun that my actual visits with doctors never entered my long-term memory, so I guess my reaction to being diagnosed with polycystic kidney disease (PKD) was met with disinterest. The only thing that disturbed me was when Mom and Dad told me I might not be able to eat salty snacks like potato chips anymore (a rule that was shortly abandoned after no doubt much whining and complaining on my part -- keep in mind, I was nine).

I also remember Mom and Dad investing in a very early and noisy water distiller. I figured it had something to do with purifying our drinking water because of Mom and I's disease, but I don't remember what it filtered out.

And that was pretty much that for the next twenty-five years. It's not that I didn't think my PKD was serious (that was hammered home to me following Mom's death at the young age of forty-one in 1992), but I simply chose not to think about it. Except for frequent migraines, I was physically healthy throughout my teens and twenties. I didn't feel any apparent effects, so I filed PKD away as an inconvenient truth that I would have to tackle at some point in the far-flung future.

That set the stage for what I consider my second diagnosis at the age of thirty-three. I had been on an ice-hiking trek in Banff, Alberta when I started to feel dizzy and disoriented. At some point, I found it hard to breathe. I got down the mountain with the help of some friendly tourists, but I still didn't feel right. I had difficulty remembering where in the Banff townsite I had parked. I found my car but lost it again after making a pit stop at a nearby McDonald's. Something was wrong, so I decided to try to find the hospital.

I was still disoriented and didn't know where to go (no cell phone GPS back then), so I stopped at a hotel to get my bearings. Some friendly Australians were working there who noticed something about me wasn't right and went out of their way to comfort me. They called the ambulance, and one very short but expensive ride later, I was at the hospital.

My disorientation was a nothing-burger and deemed to be the effects of higher elevation. However, the doctor on call was far more concerned about something that showed up in my toxicology screening. "Your kidneys aren't working too well," he said. In my mind, I pictured myself smiling, nodding and thinking, "It begins."

In retrospect, there were signs it was coming. I had started feeling increasingly worn down and frequently needed naps during my lunch break at work. But it wasn't clear to me whether that had anything to do with PKD or whether it was just the effects of being in my thirties and "getting older."

One clear symptom had been an increase in blood pressure that was bad enough for my family doctor to put me on medication (this was before I found out I was functioning on the equivalent of one kidney). I figured blood pressure was something I could control, so I targeted that with more exercise (mostly running) and avoiding salty foods. That wasn't as easy as I had thought; it was around that time that food companies started putting health information on food packaging. It was shocking how much sodium there was in even a standard loaf of bread.

After three years of meeting with nephrologists and watching my glomerular filtration rate (GFR) drop a little more every time, I was put on dialysis in May 2011. My wife and I chose home peritoneal dialysis. This type of dialysis essentially uses the membranes of the peritoneal cavity- the space between the inside of the abdomen and pelvis, at least to the best of my understanding- as a makeshift kidney. Fluid is pumped into the body and then pumped out along with the impurities the membranes have filtered. It could be done in two ways: using a machine while I was sleeping or four times a day using a manual method.

Peritoneal dialysis is a logistical nightmare. Every month, I would get boxes upon boxes of supplies. The fluid came in different strength concentrations, and I needed to decide on the kind of concentration to use based on the results from the previous day.

I did get infections on several occasions, which usually meant several days' stay in the hospital until the infection was fought back. Rinse, wash, repeat. There were good times in that period of my life of course, but I can't help but look back at those days as a particularly hellish time in my life.

Even the management of used peritoneal equipment was a never-ending struggle. The process resulted in more plastic than any renter anywhere has the garbage capacity for, especially with a bi-weekly garbage pickup. Used fluid would block up the bathroom drain and had a distinctive smell of boiled peas (and I hate boiled peas). It was a mess.

Finally, in January 2015, my nephrologist pulled some strings, securing a seat at the hemodialysis clinic in Olds, Alberta (the town between Calgary and Red Deer, where we lived at the time). The timing could not have been better; not only was the peritoneal membrane barely working by that point. Life changed virtually overnight. There was no more setting up, taking-down or management of medical supplies. I got up at 6:00 a.m., had my morning coffee, drove to the hospital about a mile away, sat in a chair and the nurses did the rest.

That's not to say it was a walk in the park. I was hooked up to a machine for four hours, three days a week. People have compared hemodialysis to running a marathon sitting down. I call that accurate because I was always exhausted by the time I was done: physically exhausted, mentally exhausted and -- for whatever reason -- depressed with a side of guilt for a little extra misery. The nurses were very good to me, and to this day, I regret that I never went back and visited them post-transplant. If any of them are reading this, please accept my humble thanks for the kindness you showed me over those three years.

Getting through the dialysis process is a matter of one day at a time. Don't look at the week with dread over all the dialysis stuff you have to do; just wake up, do what you must go to bed and start it all again the next day. Your darkest moments will come when you focus too much on the long term because the whole process, from diagnosis to transplant, can be very long.

I worked as a graphic designer at a newspaper in Olds, Alberta, and for most of the time, I was on dialysis. That experience wasn't too bad because, for all its logistical issues and infection risk, peritoneal dialysis is relatively easy on the body while it's happening. Hemodialysis is a different story. My first two months of hemodialysis coincided with my final two months at my newspaper job (my boss had decided to outsource graphic design). Every time I went to work after dialysis, I usually sat staring at my computer screen in a stupor, not knowing where to start.

The call that I had a kidney match came on the lazy Friday of March 18, 2018, and my reaction was, oddly enough, reluctance. The severity of the procedure itself had me concerned; I had already had a double nephrectomy (both kidneys were taken out because they were taking up a lot of space) just six months prior, and it was not a pleasant recovery.

Doctors and nurses have told me a reluctance to receive a kidney when one becomes available is not an uncommon reaction among transplant patients. Dialysis becomes part of one's daily or every second-day routine, and there's sometimes a sense of "It works, so why go to all that trouble to get a kidney?" Humans aren't always rational, though; we crave an emotional nest, even if that nest is made of thorns that cause us pain.

The diagnosis of PKD can seem incredibly random. Sometimes, one sibling gets it, and the other doesn't. Sometimes, the girls in a family will get it, but the boys won't, and vice versa. Sometimes, it skips an entire generation. It's an easy disease to get all "Why me?" about.

I don't criticize those who take that route because I get it. But at the same time, I wouldn't recommend it because compared to many diseases that destroy vital organs, there's hope: you can have a long life on the other side.

The immunosuppressant drugs are better than ever and are continuing to become so. In my grandmother's time, she was probably considered lucky even to get a couple of years of use out of her new kidney, while here I am, five years out from my transplant with no signs of it failing anytime soon (knock on wood).

That's my long-winded way of saying stay positive. Look after your mental health; if you're as lucky as I was, you may have a counsellor on staff in your kidney clinic who specializes in patients on dialysis. I highly recommend using their services -- they can help you learn to cope with your new reality. They also have the tools to help you find income support for whatever point you choose to stay home and off work.

I admit this is all very Canada-centric and a little

complacent in our universal health care system -- I couldn't imagine what this process would have done to my family and me if we had to pay for dialysis.

Jennifer

> *Jennifer is a granddaughter of Lily and Clarence. Her mother is Jean and her brothers are Jeremy and Justin.*

When I was young, I remember my Grandma being very sick. I didn't know why she was ill and I don't have any memory of her being anything but sick. I remember taking bus trips to Edmonton with my mom to visit my grandparents. I'm not sure how many years they had to spend in Edmonton, but I do remember them moving back to our small town.

By the time they moved back, Grandma had a

transplant by then. I remember my brother and I cuddling with her while she read us stories, but she wouldn't let my young brother sit on her right side. He was younger than me, maybe three or four, and didn't know to be careful around her right side, as that was where the transplanted kidney was. He would accidentally kick her or nudge her, and it hurt her. He was so little and just wanted to sit closer to her. I was a little older, so I was able to be more careful.

From what I recall, Grandma had some illness still, a lot of headaches, and was in the hospital frequently. Being a kid, I didn't know why; this was just how we visited Grandma. And then she was gone. I remember coming home and my mom was sitting on the floor, on the phone and crying. Grandma had passed away from complications due to a kidney transplant. I learned much later in life that she had a brain aneurysm. I didn't understand what had happened, except that my mom was upset. I recall going to my grandparents' house that same night, and everyone was crying. I was more upset to see my aunts and mom crying than a fundamental understanding of what had happened.

My next memory is again in a hospital. My mom, brother, aunt, and cousin all had ultrasounds. We all were required to check if we had cysts. We all had them. But I don't remember any genuine concern. It seemed to be a fact of life. Yes, Grandma had this; yes, we all had this. No worries. No one did much more than know about it. I don't recall any follow-up appointments or any recommendations. This condition we all had simply become a thing to know about but otherwise dismissed. I do remember, after the appointment, we went to some diner or restaurant that had a jukebox. We played 'Wasn't That a Party' by the Irish Rovers, over and over, much to the displeasure of the other patrons.

Polycystic Kidney Disease (PKD) didn't raise its head again until my Aunt passed away in a car accident. From what I understand, her final examination revealed that she was a few months away from needing dialysis. No one knew; I don't think she even knew. However, she had to have been feeling terrible. We don't know why she didn't seek any support or medical advice. When she died, it had been about twelve years since my Grandma died.

Next was my uncle; I recall he had started to fail fairly rapidly. He received a transplant and has been doing well. Then, my mom. At this point, it's been over twenty years since my Grandma passed. Again, throughout this period, there was not much mention of PKD. We mention the condition if we go to a new doctor, but there's no failure; it's still just a thing we have. How did we not think about this?

Then my cousin, then my brother, and my youngest brother all started to have renal failure. So here I am, the last one standing. I figure I made it to forty without any problems. I have cysts and kidney stones now and again. I had cysts rupture a few times, which were extremely painful events. I am a woman, so urinary tract infections are not uncommon. Despite these symptoms, for some reason, I thought it wouldn't happen to me. I figured, what are the chances? Surely, this disease would spare me; it got everyone else, and one person must remain unscathed. The doctors did say that you can live your entire life with cysts and not have a problem or experience failure. I decided I wanted that route—no such luck. I was just about forty-three when I was told that my kidneys were starting to fail. Well, hearing that, quite frankly, sucks. My kidneys had been on a downward trend for two years. The only reason I was even at the nephrologist was that I had kidney stones that wouldn't pass. Those took a year to go through (good times!)

So here I am, one of the last to hit the beginning stages of failure. I'm not going to lie; I'm scared. The reason I'm scared is not because of the unknown but because of the known--I know exactly how sick I'm going to get. I know how long it takes to wait for a kidney. I know that dialysis is extremely hard. I know my life is going to get limited and built around treatment times. Having had a significant illness once before, I can safely say I would rather not know what is going to happen.

The symptoms leading up to it are not fun either, and the kicker is that everyone has different symptoms. There isn't a textbook to follow on this one. I have fatigue, nausea, pain, infections, and stones, and I'm sure there is more to come. The brain fog that comes with fatigue is difficult to fight through. Somedays, you can feel a bit of yourself slipping away.

So, instead of facing it, I hid from it. I told my husband, of course. Then I told my boss, only because I had doctor's appointments. Then I kept quiet and went on a great holiday. I was hoping it wasn't real. But then I had another doctor's appointment. It was real; I had dropped in function again. I told my close friends. They did the appropriate thing and sympathized. However, I kept it from my children to ensure it was real. So, one appointment later, and I dropped a bit again, we decided it was time to tell the kids. Then I swore them to secrecy. I still didn't want the rest of the family to know. I am a very private person. The thought of any drama or upset doesn't sit well with me. I just want to live my life without any sort of upheaval. So here I was, feeling sicker as the year went on and not telling anyone. I'm taking naps and leaving work because I'm having lots of pain and nausea while pretending that I am just fine–eyeballing where the garbage cans are in every meeting just in case I get sick, hoping no one asks me a question while fighting to keep my breakfast down. Probably not the best way to deal with the issue. However, it's what I did.

As time went on, I realized there was no point in suffering in silence and telling people that I also have this disease is something I should do. So I told my close family, my husband's family and my immediate co-workers. All of whom were very good about it and upset that I didn't tell them sooner that I was going through this, but here we are.

I'm lucky; I'm in my forties and starting to fail. My brothers, unfortunately, started early, with the beginning of failure in their thirties. This hereditary condition is so strong that my kids also have polycystic kidneys. Even the genes of my husband were not enough to protect them. Hopefully, this does not pass on to their children.

I was off work for a bit due to the pain. I recently had one of the cysts aspirated, which is a long needle stuck through your back into the kidney cyst to drain the fluid that has accumulated in the cyst. The doctor took our seventy millilitres of fluid from a cyst about the size of a tennis ball. The relief was almost instantaneous. But it took some convincing for my doctors to consider this option. I was told that this procedure doesn't always work and the cyst fills up again anyway. I had a good six months with minimal pain, and it was totally worth it! The pain I am in is joined by fatigue, I guess it's my body's way of trying to shield me. I'm back at work with some modifications due to the fatigue but I have a great support system at home and at work who are very understanding.

I'm not even remotely close to needing dialysis. I am frustrated that the symptoms have started so early. My doctor basically said I get to be sick for a long time. Sometimes I wish my kidneys would hurry up and fail so there is some end in sight. Other times I'm grateful to be functioning as well as I am.

Jeremy

> *Jeremy is a grandson of Lily and Clarence. His mom is Jean and his siblings are Jennifer and Justin.*

The poor young lad couldn't have been more than eleven or twelve years old when he had his first ultrasound. He knew they were checking his kidneys for cysts but didn't quite have a grasp on what that meant. Let alone how the results would determine what a good portion of his life would look like.

As fate would have it, he did have cysts, but there was also something extra. As we will see, this whole 'extra wrinkle in the fabric' would become a running theme in his life. In this case, the wrinkle came in the form of kidney stones, with several in his kidneys, just chilling out, minding their business. Once again, he didn't understand the gravity of the situation, but he was pretty good at math. He devised this basic formula: Kidney + stones = pain to the power of infinity. He was scared.

It would be several years before this would manifest meaningfully, and by then, he had forgotten all about those stones. Manifest they did, though. He was seventeen years old, and pain began to course through his lower back, stomach, and groin. He had no idea what was going on. He was with his friends and, more importantly, the lady friend he was trying to impress and he didn't want to cause a scene. Silently, he powered through it. If he had known what was ailing him, he might not have been so quick to ignore it.

He would go on to have many, many more of these nasty little devils over the years. He stopped counting after twenty. Sometimes, he would power through just like the first time, and others would be in unmanageable pain. This is the story of my experience with polycystic kidney disease (PKD).

Hello. My name is Jeremy, and I am a kidney-aholic. No matter how hard I try, I simply cannot live without one. I have a little something called Polycystic Kidney Disease, or PKD for short. What happens when you have this malady involves a lot of cysts, mostly on your kidneys but also on your liver, intestines, and other assorted squishy bits. Over time, you get cysts on your cysts, and your kidneys grow until your kidneys begin to shut down. At some point, you will need either a live donor or a deceased donor and will need dialysis while you wait. PKD is a tricky beast, though. It's a genetic condition, and it runs strong in my family. A live donor, while typically the best option, is unlikely for me since pretty much everyone in my family has this condition. Complicating matters further, I have a rare blood type, so finding a kidney was even more difficult. Realistically, dialysis was my only real option and I had a choice between peritoneal or hemodialysis when my blood scrubbers (a.k.a. kidneys) gave up the ghost.

When given the option, I chose to do the peritoneal route for my dialysis. To understand how this works, you need to know what the peritoneal cavity is. The most straightforward description is that a sack inside you contains your intestines, stomach, liver and spleen. The walls of the sack are ultrathin and absorbent. A catheter is surgically implanted into that sack and used to fill that cavity with a special fluid. This fluid leeches impurities out of the peritoneal walls, partially doing the kidneys' job. After the catheter is implanted, it takes a long time to heal, about nine months. Because of this extended healing period, they put the entire thing under your skin, only pulling the end out when you are about to start using it.

Now that the general explanation is out of the way, this is where my story begins. The morning I was to start dialysis, I went to the hospital to have my catheter "externalized." I was led into a small side room by a doctor. He lifted my t-shirt and injected my stomach area with a numbing agent to prevent pain. Then he cut me open. While I could feel him fishing around inside me, his cell phone rang, and Sandstorm by DaRude was his ringtone. Not only did he get a call while performing minor surgery, he answered it. I think he was making lunch plans with someone.

Dr. Sandstorm started getting a little frustrated after some more yanking and tugging. He kept commenting about how deep and stubborn my catheter was. His phone rang again; you'd think he would turn off the ringer after that first faux pas, but no. This time, he didn't answer. He couldn't decline the call either, as he was knuckles deep in my guts, so we got to hear practically the whole song as he continued to work.

One short eternity later, he was done. My next step was to walk over to the building across the street where the actual peritoneal clinic was. Okay, off I go. By the time I arrived at the clinic, the freezing was starting to wear off, and things were starting to hurt. The icing on this tragic cake was that Dr. Sandstorm didn't even bandage me up, so my t-shirt was soaked with blood by the time I got there.

As the months went by, every time I would report to the clinic, they would note that I was not getting enough clearance [not enough of the blood was being cleaned], and they would strengthen the dose of the fluid I would have to use. It got to the point where the fluid was so strong I was constantly breaking out in little red spots all over my body. The reaction was so intense that the nurse was skeptical that I was doing dialysis at all. It seems my peritoneal lining was just not absorbent enough to get the cleaning I needed not to die—time to move on to hemodialysis.

This type of dialysis is the kind most are familiar with. You go to the hospital, get hooked up to a machine for four hours, and then go home exhausted and freezing. Of course, before this, I needed another surgery to create a fistula, a special network of veins that are structured to have enough blood flow for the hemodialysis machine to work properly. Typically the fistula would be put in the forearm, unfortunately in my case, nothing is normal. They discovered that the veins in my forearms were no good, and they had to put the fistula in my bicep instead. To develop the network of veins to be effective, I had to lift tiny five-pound weights with that arm constantly.

After my arm healed and I could start hemodialysis, I had to have yet another surgery, to get that peritoneal catheter out of my guts. Oddly, it went off without a hitch, and I was thankful for it. In the first few weeks of hemodialysis, you learn that everybody reacts differently to the process. Some people feel great after and can go to work a regular eight-hour shift when they are done. Some people get sick, some get allergic reactions, and some get incredibly exhausted. My reaction was exhaustion and migraines–three sessions a week, three migraines a week. I would come home from dialysis and just lay in a blacked-out room, wishing the building would collapse on my face.

After about a year of this, the doctors found a medicine that would counteract the migraines if I took it just before I started my treatment. This medicine was a lifesaver as I spent four years on dialysis. I had to survive on dialysis longer than most because, of course, I have a rare blood type, which made finding a donor kidney more difficult.

The thing I never expected about hemodialysis

was the emotional toll it took on me. I was assigned to the dialysis unit at the Edmonton General Hospital, which is now a giant palliative care center. Almost everyone around me was old, lonely, sad, and dying. A massive room full of human misery. Every nurse who worked there must have been superhuman because this experience ate away at my soul.

Being called in as a backup when a kidney becomes available is not unusual. A deceased donor usually has two kidneys. The transplant team would call in three people just in case someone was disqualified, which was not uncommon. What is unusual is being called in as backup six times. All the nurses in the transplant unit said they'd never seen anyone come in as a backup more than twice. I smashed that record, baby! The seventh and final call came at 4:00 a.m. one weekend in November, less than twelve hours after the sixth call. I didn't even believe them.

According to what I've been told, the procedure was fraught with peril. I was unconscious for most of it. The surgery was supposed to take four hours, but it ran closer to seven. I remember half a dozen nurses standing around me, yelling for me to wake up. I guess it was getting touch-and-go for a while as to whether I would wake up at all. My family was told the new kidney was initially working fine, but it was not when I was deposited back in my room. It slowly started to kick in over the next few days. I think it's safe to say my new kidney was a bit of an underachiever. I spent seven days in the hospital. Nurses and doctors filtered in and out of my room, fussing about one thing or another. They had me up and walking the very next morning after the procedure. I had never felt so weak in my entire life; putting one foot in front of the other was a herculean task. I persevered, and they let me out into the wild after a week.

The next few weeks after the surgery were by far the most difficult days I've experienced in my entire life. It's mostly just a blur of pain, exhaustion, naps, and trips to the hospital for tests. At one point, I was wishing I never had the surgery. Apparently, at the time, I thought a lifetime in a soul-crushing dialysis chair was preferable. Slowly, it got better.

Before I had the transplant, I had heard that

some people would get odd and unsettling feelings upon getting a donor organ. It would be described as thoughts and feelings that were not their own. It is almost as if the foreign body part somehow could exert some of the original owner's traits on its host. I brushed it off as silly nonsense until it happened to me. It's a purely psychological thing, it's unsettling, to say the least.

Six weeks after the transplant, there was supposed to be a minor procedure where they yank a little silicone brace out of your new kidney connection from your urethra. The brace is left in during the operation to help the connection between your new kidney and your bladder heal properly (it's even more fun than it sounds). My surgeon decided to bump my appointment up to four weeks after the surgery. He went on vacation directly after, which may or may not have factored into his decision. After he was done, he tried to console me. Telling me that although it is a truly awful experience, at least it only has to be done once.

A few weeks later, the pain started. I had a sharp stabbing pain whenever I moved around the new kidney area. When I reported it to my nurses, they brushed it off as me trying to do too much too soon. They advised more rest. I had a feeling it was something much worse, so I wouldn't let it go. At last, they begrudgingly decided to ultrasound the area. I was only halfway home from the hospital after the scan when I got a call from them. I needed to come back to the hospital right away, and I needed to be booked in for surgery ASAP. In a fantastic coincidence, the area where the little silicone brace was had necrotized and was dead, almost like it was taken out too early. The area was also completely crusted over with hardened calcium. The plan was laparoscopic surgery. They were going to go in and remove all the calcium. When I woke up from the operation, the doctor came in with the good news and the bad news. The good news was that the calcium was gone. The bad news was that the whole area was dead. The actual part that was dead was the tube from the kidney to the bladder. Put another way, there was no path for urine to move from my kidney to my bladder. I would have to wear a plastic bag strapped to my leg for urine to drain out from until they could get me in to essentially re-do my original transplant.

The third surgery I found to be even worse than the first one. It was the same procedure, with the added complication of the drain bag and an extra hole in my side. The big difference is that I had so many people come and support me during my transplant. It fed me the energy and will to push forward, but I had very few visitors this second time. Depression and despair were my greatest enemies at this time. I had sworn I never wanted to go through transplant surgery again, and here I was three months later, doing exactly that.

I then had several complications. The fistula that I had on my arm developed an aneurysm and slowly worsened in the last few years until it needed to be removed. The pain in my arm proceeded to get much, much worse. The worst pain I have ever felt in my life. The nurse and several doctors waved it off as not a big deal, but I knew it was something more serious. It turns out the pain was caused by a severe blood clot from the wrist to the shoulder. I was within days of losing the entire limb. This time, when I woke up from the operation, there were three surgeons gathered around and as they were talking, my hand started to ache badly. As fate would have it, zero blood flowed into my hand. I then needed another surgery. I had only gotten one bite of my waffle breakfast.

After the third operation, in less than a month, I had about half of the amount of blood flowing through my arm that I should have. The surgical team offered to try a fourth time, but I called it good enough there. I was already facing a lifetime of pain in my arm from all the damage done. I didn't trust them to get the job done properly.

It's been a few years now, and I wish there were a happy ending. Unfortunately, I struggle with dangerously low iron and dangerously high potassium. There are so many things your kidneys are supposed to regulate and control. Chronic pain and exhaustion are a daily struggle. As are depression, guilt, uncertainty, and a general sense of existential dread. At my relatively young age, I will almost certainly need a second transplant. Replacement kidneys don't last forever.

Typically kidneys are supposed to 'activate'

vitamin D, causing your body to absorb calcium. However, my transplanted kidney is not doing what it should be and is causing hyperparathyroidism (one or more of the parathyroid glands in your neck produce too much parathyroid hormone), which in turn means that I have to have my parathyroid glands removed, which, of course, means more surgery. A surgery that risks damaging my vocal cords. After that procedure, I'll tell you all about it, if I can. It never ends.

As they say, there is no cure for kidney disease. There are only treatments, and a transplant is a treatment. I, and many other victims of faulty kidneys, will continue to struggle with a myriad of assorted complications for our entire lives. It's a battle with no end or reprieve against an enemy that cannot be defeated. I've often been asked, "How?" How do you deal with it day in and day out? By realizing I have no choice. I don't know how often I have said, "I can't anymore." I've been wrong every single time so far. My strategy is to continue being wrong whenever I say, "I can't."

Justin

> *Justin is a grandson of Lily and Clarence. His mom is Jean and his siblings are Jennifer and Jeremy.*

As a child, I don't recall talking as a family about kidney disease. I recall it being very hush-hush. I remember hearing the adults talking about my mom's hospital visits. And how Grandma died from the disease. And how sick Aunt Donna was. As an adult, I've had a few good conversations with my brother and my mom about our experiences. I always got the impression that nobody wanted to acknowledge that we had this family disease. It's like if we ignore it, it will go away.

When I was diagnosed, I didn't know much about what I was in for. I knew so little that I went to a family doctor to see if I could donate to Mom. He laughed and said, *"You realize you have the same disease, right?"* So, I chose the 'ignore it' method. I just carried on with my life until I started getting actual symptoms.

I didn't get a whole lot of symptoms until I got closer to being considered in kidney failure, which is below forty percent. I've been tired and worn out, yet sleeping is challenging. As the failure started, I began to have symptoms such as extreme anxiety, restless legs, brain fog, depression and lots of kidney stones.

To manage the symptoms, I used to try to numb myself with drugs and alcohol. Now, I find there isn't much I can do about the physical pain except just deal with it. Tough it out. The mental issues, I just try to find ways to keep my mind busy, whether it's work, the kids, or things to do around the house.

I don't know what kind of advice to offer,

everybody is different and has different support systems. Don't let doctors and nurses walk all over you. Be an advocate for yourself or have someone who can speak up on your behalf. Don't ever let anyone invalidate your feelings. Nobody knows how you are feeling except you, and I find that to be the hardest part. We don't look sick for the most part. Even our partners can forget sometimes. Don't take it to heart, even though it can be hard sometimes.

Remember that you aren't alone. There are so many support groups. Talk to family and friends. Make them aware. Do research. Don't be afraid to ask questions, no matter how insignificant you think they may be. Don't hide your condition from your kids. They need to know what to expect.

End of the Story...sort of

Well, this is where we are today in our journey with Autosomal Dominant Polycystic Kidney Disease. Our story isn't over; some of us are still travelling down the well-worn path of this illness. This chronicle was never intended as a "feel sorry for us" diatribe and was not intended to scare anyone. We want to demonstrate that this disease leads to a complicated path that affects everyone, even family members, so differently. No guidebook or textbook will tell you what you feel is normal. We share so others in the same situation know they are not alone; we hear you.

This disease takes a toll on you physically and mentally in a never-ending circle, not just on you but on your support system as well. Try to live your life as normally as you can. Take that trip you've been putting off, go to school, change jobs, take skydiving lessons, or do whatever it is you think you can't do. Do it anyway. If you have polycystic kidney disease, the illness is going to come whether you wish it or not, so take advantage of the moments you feel good.

Remember, there are people just like you, and help is available. Make sure your support system is in place and use it. That's what people who care about you want to do–be there for you through thick and thin.

Frequently Asked Questions

Much information has been shared in It's All Relative, but we may have yet to answer many questions. While not an exhaustive list, this FAQ attempts to address some oddities with kidney disease. Some of these are my questions, and others I have heard. Take what you will from the information provided.

Why am I craving ice chips?

A little research has revealed an actual name for this: Pica. It's a craving for non-nutritional substances. Though it is a named issue, there is not a lot of research on it in terms of kidney disease, though there is mention that it could be related to an iron deficiency, which is always possible with kidney disease. I'm told when you're in a dialysis clinic, they go through ice chips like gangbusters. Ice chips are also common to crave when nauseous. The cool of the ice seems to help and is not a foreign substance.

Why am I so thirsty?

So far, I can't find a clear answer. Still, the kidneys appear to lose the capacity to concentrate urine, which means that the kidneys use more water from your body to remove solutes, which in turn makes you thirsty, thus drinking more to replace the lost fluid.

Does PKD brain fog and perimenopause brain fog collide?

So far, I can't find any studies on this, nor do my doctors think that this is real. But living with it right now, I can tell one or the other or both make brain fog a terrible thing to live through. I assume fatigue with the disease doesn't help, either. But if you can recognize it for what it is, at least you can spend some time developing some strategies to help yourself. I will say that any woman of our particular generational vintage, take heart – you're not the only one!

I'm losing my hair. Can that happen?

From what I'm told, the stress of dialysis and possibly some of the medications with treatment or dialysis may be causing the hair loss. A good hairdresser can help with that, as can some shampoos. The stress of the disease can contribute to the loss of hair. Any extreme stress may cause hair loss, even if you do not have a chronic illness.

My doctor says I shouldn't feel any pain with polycystic kidneys, so why is there pain?

If you feel pain, the pain is real. Everything is connected, and while it might not originate in your kidney, it could be the kidney pressing on something else. All that pressure could be causing some pain.

I'm having weird symptoms, but my doctor says it's not connected to kidney disease. What should I do?

Well, maybe it is, and perhaps it isn't. I've learned in this journey that there is no "normal." You have to be your advocate. There isn't anyone watching you closely to make sure you are okay. If you feel off, talk to your family doctor and your nephrologist. Then, push for whatever else you need. But please don't ask Dr. Interweb!

Can cysts rupture or pop?

Though an accurate diagnosis of a ruptured cyst can only be made through diagnostic testing, you can feel a cyst rupture. For me, it starts similar to flu-like symptoms, feeling like a bit of fever and nausea. Then the pain begins, like a stone, but not as bad. Once it pops, you feel the relief spreading through your body. When you go to the restroom, there may be some black flecks and an oily sheen in the toilet.

Why do I feel guilty for receiving a kidney?

To be honest, I'm not there yet, but I can imagine that it's because of the knowledge that someone had to die for you to live. A family lost a loved one who was gracious enough to donate their organs to help another person. It may also be survivor's guilt that you got the kidney and someone else did not. Please make sure to talk to someone about how you are feeling to maintain your mental health. And remember, this is a good thing for you and will improve.

Is there support for people with kidney disease?

If you live in Canada, the Kidney Foundation is a not-for-profit organization that helps kidney patients locate the information and resources they need to learn more about managing kidney disease.

Is there support after you receive a transplant?

There is a medical team for technical support, but emotional support is harder to find. I haven't found too many support groups or places to ask questions to help manage some of the emotions that appear to come with receiving a transplant. I suggest you advocate for yourself, find counselling or set up a support network and invite others to join.

What can I do to help further study kidney disease and its effects?

If you're willing, you can join drug trials, focus groups or complete surveys to answer questions about your health and life with kidney disease. I've joined Kidney Link, a research platform searching for patients to participate in various studies.

I'm still at a reasonably high function. Others in healthcare always tell me I'm fine, but I don't feel fine. Is that okay?

You feel how you feel. Some have no symptoms, some have many, and others swing in between. There is no normal. Depending on your rate of decline, you could feel symptoms for a very long time. Take heart; there are others out there that feel the same. Please know there is nothing wrong with feeling sick at a high function.

Acknowledgements

Thank you to my family for being so willing to be vulnerable. I can't imagine it was easy for them to share their innermost thoughts and feelings. For me, this was an interesting exploration into my own family. I learned so much from their accounts that I might otherwise have never known. I learned more than I've ever known about my Grandmother, shining such a bright light on everything she went through with her illness.

This was a hard story to write and even harder to share. My family and I have opened up to the world and now I feel exposed but the point is to be vulnerable, sharing the hard journeys we have travelled to help others know they are not alone.

References

Kidney Foundation - The Kidney Foundation of Canada - Home Page, https://kidney.ca/. Accessed 27 February 2024.

KidneyLink – Connecting Canadians to kidney research, 28 April 2023, https://kidneylink.ca/. Accessed 27 February 2024.

"Kidneys: Location, Anatomy, Function & Health." *Cleveland Clinic*, 17 May 2022, https://my.clevelandclinic.org/health/body/21824-kidney. Accessed 27 February 2024.

"Kidney stones - Symptoms, causes, types,

and treatment." *National Kidney Foundation*, https://www.kidney.org/atoz/content/kidneystones. Accessed 27 February 2024.

"What is ADPKD?" *PKD Foundation*, https://pkdcure.org/what-is-adpkd/. Accessed 27 February 2024.

Dugdale, David C., and Brenda Conaway. "Hyperparathyroidism - Symptoms and Causes." *Penn Medicine*, https://www.pennmedicine.org/for-patients-and-visitors/patient-information/conditions-treated-a-to-z/hyperparathyroidism. Accessed 23 April 2024.

Journal of Clinical Sleep Medicine. "Restless Legs Syndrome in Non-Dialysis Renal Patients: Is It Really That Common?" *Journal of Clinical Sleep Medicine*, vol. 11, no. 1, 2015, p. 1. *Journal of Clinical Sleep Medicine*, https://jcsm.aasm.org/doi/10.5664/jcsm.4366. Accessed 30 04 2024.

National Human Genome Research Institute. "About Autosomal Dominant Polycystic Kidney Disease." *National Human Genome Research Institute*, 18 April 2013, https://www.genome.gov/Genetic-Disorders/Autosomal-Polycystic-Kidney-Disease. Accessed 1 May 2024.

Urology Care Foundation. "Kidney Failure: Symptoms, Causes & Diagnosis." *Urology Care Foundation*, https://www.urologyhealth.org/urology-a-z/k/kidney-(renal)-failure. Accessed 1 May 2024.

Pleura and Peritoneum. "Morphology of the peritoneal cavity and pathophysiological consequences." *Pleura and Peritoneum*, vol. 1, no. 4, 2016, p. 1. *De Gruyter Brill*, https://www.degruyter.com/document/doi/10.1515/pp-2016-0023/html?lang=en. Accessed 5 5 2024.

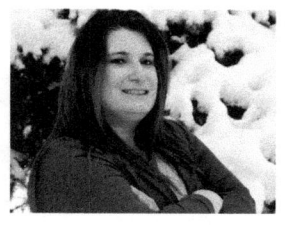

Jennifer Florax always states that her writing is founded on her life experiences, with a strong desire to impart valuable lessons to others to help them avoid unnecessary pain and expedite their learning curve. Jennifer emphasizes that she is not an expert but a knowledgeable individual who shares hard-earned lessons and years of experience gained in diverse environments.

Other books by Jennifer Florax

The Hunt: The Job Of Finding Employment

The Hunt breaks down the search for a job as an employee and provides an overview from the employer's perspective, providing straight-to-the-point tips to assist in finding a job. Knowing what an employer is looking for will help you tailor your résumé to a potential employer's needs. Advice for both perspectives is the same: set a goal, identify what you need, be selective, and put in the work.

Survival Guide for the Working World: What School Doesn't Teach You

We spend a significant amount of time and investment ensuring that our young people are fully versed in the technical requirements of work life. We assume (wrongfully) that they are born into understanding the acceptable work norms or behaviours - what we in the work world call 'soft skills.' Survival

Guide for the Working World offers tips, tricks and bite-sized bits of the workforce, including how to dress, write an email, perspective seeking, the value of a mentor, and customer service, to name a few topics.

Printed in the USA
CPSIA information can be obtained
at www.ICGtesting.com
LVHW010223310724
786664LV00011B/535